FORGETIQUETTE

*What to do when someone
you love begins to forget*

JOAN SAUERS

BANTAM
SYDNEY AUCKLAND TORONTO NEW YORK LONDON

For the unforgettable Don Sauers and Ted Heery

All relationships are hard, but when someone you love has dementia that relationship (and your sanity!) can be even harder to maintain. Over the years my once quick-witted father gradually lost his memory, and the strain on his caregivers was excruciating. As he neared the end of his life, my wonderful father-in-law also started to lose touch with the here and now. Both have passed away, and I miss them every day. Although it wasn't easy, I did find ways to cope with the confusing, awkward and sometimes heartbreaking situations that arose when dementia struck, and I've tried to distil them in this book. Thankfully, there are simple things you can do to get through it with grace and dignity. So, cut yourself some slack and remember that common sense, humour and love will go a long way.

Leave your pedantry and control-freakiness at the door. Because, so far, dementia is incurable. And even though treatments for Alzheimer's and other forms of the disease are different, the etiquette of dealing with them is the same.

First, change the way you think about people becoming senile. Try not to see it as tragic. Deep down, they're still the person you love. Just remember that *you'll* have to adapt to *their* changes, not the other way around.

Talk about dementia before it comes calling. Hiding it in the closet neither prevents it from coming nor makes it go away. Ultimately, giving it some light and air makes it easier to deal with.

A sense of humour will be your salvation.

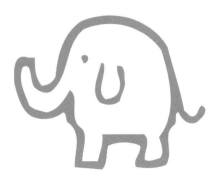

If your parent or partner suspects they have dementia, take them to get checked out pronto. Early diagnosis will give them the best tools to cope.

And ask for advice about how to handle things yourself.

Which, trust me, won't be easy.

Very rarely will someone admit they can't look after themselves, so it's important to watch for telltale signs.

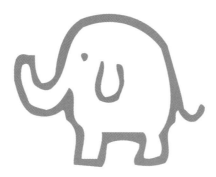

Like their sunglasses in the fridge. Or the cat in the microwave.

If *you* suspect a loved one has dementia but they're in denial, gently help them to recognise that it might be getting harder for them to balance their budget. Or remember what the toaster is for.

You might be surprised at their relief when they can admit what's happening.

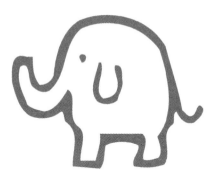

Whether they want to go or not, get them to a doctor.

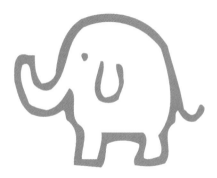

Loss of balance can be an early indicator that they might be at risk.

Talk about dementia without judgement. The stigma is what keeps people from accepting they have it.

And don't be afraid to be upbeat and even funny! Who cares if it's in questionable taste if it makes your old man smile?

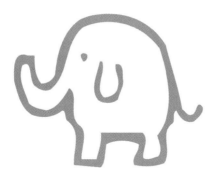

Dementia can be masked when the sufferer has always been dominated by their partner. If mum has always worn the pants, then who's to notice when dad can't put his on by himself?

If dementia is confirmed early, you can talk about what *they* want while they still have some of their marbles.

But don't write them off too soon! Many people have only mild symptoms for years and can get away with excusing the odd senior moment as 'normal'. Whatever that is. In the meantime, you can use their insight into their own illness to help *you* help *them*.

Get her to a lawyer who specialises in Elder Law before mum is too far gone to make end-of-life decisions for herself. The less you have to decide on your own down the line, the better.

Dad's condition will worsen faster if you do everything for him.

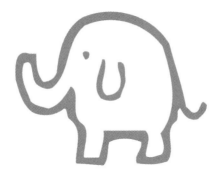

If he wants to, let him make his own sandwich, even if it takes him an hour and a half and the kitchen ends up looking like a crime scene.

When they say their memory is gone, tell them they've achieved what Zen Buddhists strive for: living in the moment!

Five minutes later when they say their memory is gone, tell them about the Zen Buddhists all over again.

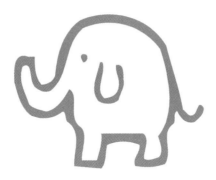

They can become agitated for what seems like no reason, but there is *always* a reason if you can find it. They might be hot or cold or need to pee – eventually your powers of deduction will triumph. But if not, distract them and they might just forget what was bugging them.

Remember that shame is contagious. If you're ashamed about their condition, they'll feel it too.

Even if they act like a seven-year-old, don't treat them like one.
They're not children; they're adults with memory loss.

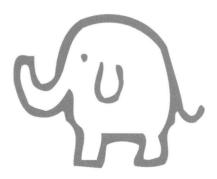

And remember, they haven't suddenly become stupid.

Just forgetful.

Dementia has been linked to a history of trauma, so be especially vigilant with victims of post-traumatic stress disorder.

Surround them with pictures of their childhood homes and loved ones.

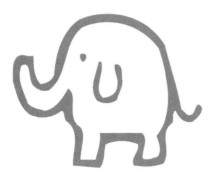

Play them some Golden Oldies. Their favourite songs will give them a sense of their place in life's narrative.

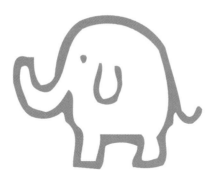

Or hook them up to YouTube with some big, comfy headphones so they can watch *and* listen to the Glenn Miller Orchestra play 'Moonlight Serenade'.

If the sufferer is your partner, you might enjoy listening to this blast from the past together. And remember that music offers pleasures and connections verging on the mystical.

Music is also proven to calm people with dementia during stressful activities, such as meals and bath time. As long as it's music *they* like, so keep your death metal playlist to yourself.

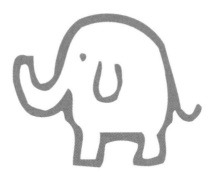

One of the quirks of dementia is that while recent memories fade, older ones can linger. So, listen as they take you on a guided tour of the past, even if the details are a bit bogus. If your mum thinks she went on that trip to Paris with Cary Grant instead of your father, does it really matter?

As in dreams, the person they imagine (Cary Grant) is simply
a representation of the real thing (your dad).
So, cut them some slack!

Unintentional slights to loved ones are inevitable and must be forgiven. On the spot.

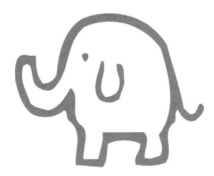

Accept that you will occasionally feel hurt. And then man up and deal with it.

Think of it as the circle of cognitive life. They started out as babies not having a clue how to look after themselves, but gradually they learned.

And now they're unlearning.

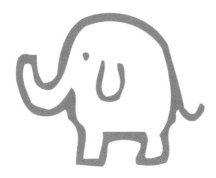

And if your once mild-mannered husband reaches the stage of a two-year-old, remember that stubbornness and tantrums are simply his way of asserting his individuality.

Find ways to blow off steam – other than in their face. Looking after people who forget can be maddening, but it won't do them or *you* any good to rub their noses in it.

Label everyday things when they start getting confused. The fridge, the kettle and the TV might have self-evident functions to you, but in the mind of a dementia sufferer they can become telephones or hair dryers or alien spacecraft.

And remember that positive reinforcement works just as well on them as it does on any of us.

Never say, 'I already told you that!' If they remembered you already told them that, they wouldn't be asking again.

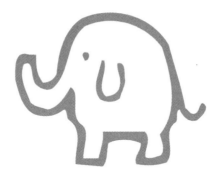

Don't bust them when they pretend to remember something they obviously don't. They may have lost their memory, but don't make them lose their dignity.

Remove clutter from the home, especially if an object's function is confusing. Like the Italian multi-head espresso machine they got five years ago for Christmas, and couldn't work out how to use even then!

But never get rid of favourite things, no matter how pointless or trivial they seem to you. Anything with sentimental value can be a magical touchstone for them.

Take locks off bathroom and bedroom doors so you can help them if necessary.

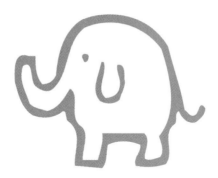

But install locks on outside windows and doors. Your dad may not have been a nudist gypsy in his youth, but you'll be amazed how often he'll enjoy ending up naked at the police station now.

When you can't take it anymore, go into the bathroom and scream into a towel. Follow that with a shot of Scotch.

And give *them* an occasional drink unless other health issues forbid it. Just because they've lost their memory doesn't mean they can't have fun!

Don't continually correct them when they get things wrong. This will only feed their fears and insecurities.

Use a day-of-the-week pill box. Even if they claim to remember taking their medication, you'll need to check.

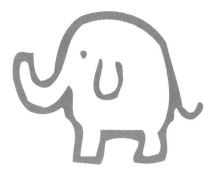

If you haven't heard of adult day care, get into it. A few hours' break can be a lifesaver for *both* of you, and keep them socialised and alert for longer.

Become a master of the bait and switch. They can act like a three-year-old on the first morning of day care when separated from their primary carer, so be ready with clever distractions.

Put childproof latches on kitchen and bathroom cabinets you
don't want them to get into . . .

Unless you want them to sprinkle drain cleaner on their cornflakes.

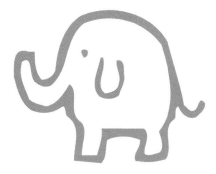

Be prepared for 'sundowning' – the phenomenon whereby they get more antsy and paranoid when the sun goes down. Experts are not sure why this happens, but the fact is you may have to persuade granny that her nice neighbour isn't actually a Nazi operative trying to poison the dog.

Read up on the science of the disease. When you understand concepts like brain shrinkage and atrophy, you'll better understand why your wife, who once lectured in particle physics, has no idea how to tell the time.

It may seem pointless to tell them good news because they'll just forget it, but it's not. Good news will trigger happy hormones, so the good vibes will linger even if the reason is forgotten.

If you have some bad news, consider not passing it along. They'll only forget it and then you'll have to tell them all over again. Do they really need to experience the pain of hearing repeatedly that their dog/son/wife/best friend has pancreatic cancer?

Keep a notebook dedicated to their care, with doctors' names, meds, phone numbers, medical history and dietary requirements. That way, you'll only have to grab one thing if you have to rush to hospital.

Before you think you'll need to access them, organise their files, including tax, insurance, wills, banking, etc. That way, when you *do* need them you'll know where to look and you won't have to wade through paperwork going back fifty years.

The more they forget, the more they will fabricate memories. But instead of challenging them, accept that this is their way of trying to embed themselves in the story – *any* story! – of their life.

And remember that most of our memories are unreliable anyway.

Even without dementia.

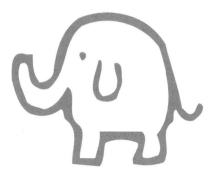

Pay them compliments. Even if you're lying. When you counteract their growing sense of inadequacy, you can lift their mood. And yours!

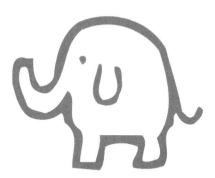

Let them play with kids. The younger the company, the less likely it is they will be judged.

Show them photo albums in chronological order and tell them the story of their life. It's fun to watch them be amazed by their own achievements and adventures.

And the bad hair they had in the 70s.

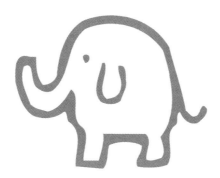

No matter how accepting *you* are, people with memory loss might try to hide it because they see it as a personality flaw. Don't buy into this. Help them accept themselves.

Even as it gets worse, don't treat their dementia like a dirty family secret. Everyone will feel better if you treat their condition as part of the wallpaper.

Get them to wear some ID or a medical bracelet in case they go walkabout.

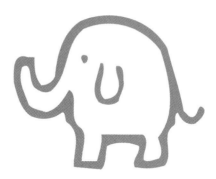

Often, one of the most distressing things for someone with dementia is to have to stop driving, an activity that symbolises freedom, fun and access to the world. So, once they start parking a little too creatively or running over the neighbour's dog, get their doctor to tell them it's on his or her orders. Don't *you* be the one to take their licence away or they may never forgive you.

When they repeat things over and over again, remember they're not trying to be annoying. They can't help it!

When they repeat things over and over again, make a game of altering your own responses slightly to keep from dying of boredom. Or strangling them.

Or when you have to tell them the same thing over and over, treat it like a mantra – a repeated phrase that could have salutary effects.

When you have to take them to the doctor or some other appointment, don't tell them until an hour or so before it's time.

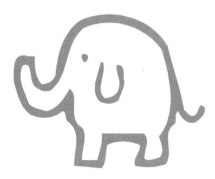

And bring along something to distract them, like a snack or a drink or some photos on your phone they may enjoy.

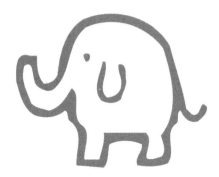

And remember that anything that keeps *them* happy,

keeps *you* happy.

Never use the word 'remember' with them. It will be a constant reminder that they *don't* remember.

Include them in group conversations even if they can't keep up. A sense of inclusion – even illusory – is vital to their wellbeing.

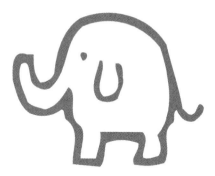

And if you forget what being marginalised feels like, try to remember your first day at a new school, or not being picked for the team or invited to a party.

Memory loss doesn't make them invalids. So, take them out for walks, especially to places like parks and beaches. Nature has a wonderful way of making you *both* feel better.

People with dementia love long drives. The passing scenery both stimulates and soothes.

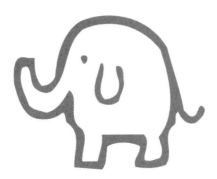

In fact, take them out as much as possible, as long as you don't lose them along the way.

Install grab bars and a non-skid mat in the shower. They can forget what they're doing right in the middle of doing it, and it's good to give them something to hold on to as they try to re-orientate themselves.

Don't be surprised if your mum can't remember what a hairbrush is for but can recite the entire *Rubáiyát of Omar Khayyám*. Memory loss can be weirdly selective.

If it's your partner whose memory is failing, seek out extra support. You're probably no spring chicken yourself and caring for him can be exhausting.

Enlist your family's help. You'll need it. Who knows?
It might bring you closer together.

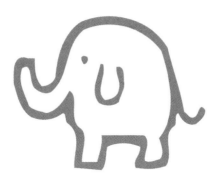

You may not like being the bad cop, but occasionally you will have to be. Tough love was never so tough, so make sure you have people around who make *you* feel good about yourself at the end of the day.

Fresh sensory stimuli will keep them engaged and happy, even if they don't know where the hell they are or what the hell they're doing there. So, get them to help you decorate the cake or wash the car or fold the laundry. Even if they don't do it perfectly, they will enjoy the simple act of doing. And doing it with you. Just don't over-stimulate, which can make them anxious.

If he has a favourite outfit, consider buying several sets. And if that happens to be a Spiderman suit, who cares – he's *ninety!* Let his freak flag fly. Arrange the clothes in the order they're meant to be put on so he can move through the process smoothly.

And opt for elastic waists and Velcro instead of buttons and zippers. This is where the superhero outfit is beginning to make sense, right?

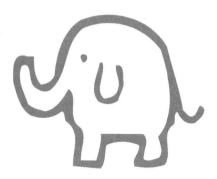

A peculiar side-effect of dementia can be a penchant for deconstructing words, so don't be surprised if they start punning and exercising some strange wordplay. Play along with them!

Obsessive hoarding of things without value is a favourite pastime of dementia sufferers, so if you want to eliminate twenty years' worth of newspapers and junk mail, do it gradually, and while they're asleep.

Even if mum always liked you best, enlist the help of siblings when she needs wrangling.

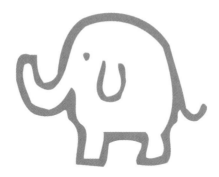

If you're an only child, ask your partner, your kids, the postman or anyone you can to help you look after her. This is not a job anyone can do alone. And enjoy your newfound skills as a delegator.

Remember, one day it might be *you* forgetting where you put your slippers (and that they don't hang from your ears), so be even more patient than you think you can be.

Unless you forget.

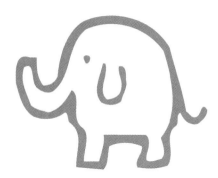

Watch some of their favourite old movies with them. Even if they can't follow the plot, it will resonate on some deep subterranean level when Bacall says to Bogart, 'If you want me, just whistle.'

Even if they make a bit of a mess when they eat, try to keep them at the family table. Anything that isolates a dementia sufferer will make their condition worse.

They can have days when they know you and days when they don't, but don't take it personally – it's the nature of the beast.

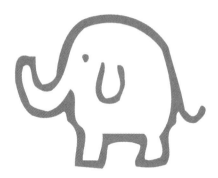

Don't try to *talk* them into remembering stuff they remembered yesterday. Memory isn't a matter of will.

The moment their dementia is first diagnosed, help them get brain rehabilitation therapy. Just as with stroke victims, early treatment may actually slow their decline.

Write letters to your member of parliament, the minister for health and any rich people you know to support the search for a cure. Discoveries are being made all the time, but you want the cure to get here before *you* start forgetting where the toothpaste goes.

Give yourself a break. 24/7 care of dementia sufferers can drive you crazy long before your own senility kicks in.

If it won't add to your burden, get them a pet. Dogs and cats are proven to keep them happy, engaged and even healthier for longer.

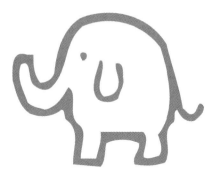

Find out what sort of in-home care is available. Nursing homes are a last resort. But when the time comes, don't beat yourself up about removing them from their own home or not keeping them at home with you.

If they're in care and you suspect they're not being treated right, do something about it. Dementia patients can be soft targets for bullies and thugs.

If they're in earshot, don't talk to others as if they aren't there.
They have dementia; they're not invisible.

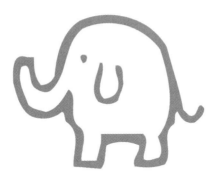

If he's struggling to find the right word, give him a chance to find it before gently offering what the word might be.

As the disease progresses, use simple words and short sentences. But *never* talk to them in a baby voice.

If your mum clings to a doll she believes is you as a baby, let her. What's important isn't what's real, but what she *believes* is real.

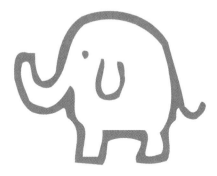

While they're still in their own home but unable to cook for themselves, discover Meals on Wheels – the greatest invention of modern man. Use them. Thank them. Put them in your will.

Mum might think the woman you've hired to clean her flat is scary or intrusive; on the other hand, she might like her better than she likes you! But don't feel hurt. Sometimes strangers are easier because they come baggage-free. And enjoy the break a stranger can give you.

Hallucinations are common, so if your dad suddenly starts acting like a toddler on acid, don't tell him he's imagining it. It's real to *him*, and all part of the whacky world of dementia.

And if he starts acting/dressing/talking like Mick Jagger, let him. He may even be quite sure he *is* Mick Jagger, but don't contradict him. Have you ever seen them in the same room?

Don't make her promise to take her pills or brush her teeth or not go outside alone. Promising doesn't make it easier to remember. But it might make her feel worse when she realises she's broken a promise.

What looks like a loony fixation to you may just be them trying to do something they don't realise they've already done. Like putting their night cream on for the seventeenth time.

Or they might start fixating on things that seem to make no sense —
having enough tinned peaches or keeping the fan on all day and night
or wearing only one worn-out pair of shoes.

What makes no sense to you might make perfect sense to them, so don't sweat anything that doesn't put them in danger.

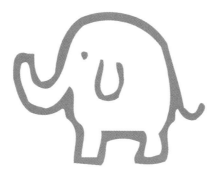

Encourage them to drink coffee – a proven memory booster.

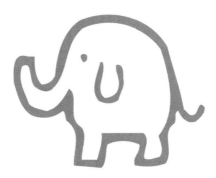

To make sure you have his attention, call the dementia sufferer by his name before you start talking to him. Hearing his name also reinforces his sense of self. Give him enough time to answer and try not to interrupt.

Join a gym or take up power walking – the frustration of caring for them can take a physical toll, and it's better to pound a punching bag than grandad.

Don't be surprised if mum gets really clingy when you leave her.

She doesn't remember when you'll be back or if you'll *ever* be back.

So, be as casual and reassuring as you can.

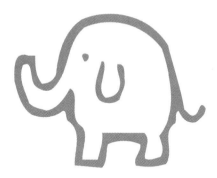

As the dementia advances, it may get harder to show them great love, but that's when they need it most.

Before their memory goes completely, they may be caught in the worst part of the disease: when they feel they should know where they are, what they're doing and who they're with, but in truth they're clueless. So, you may need to tell them what's happening as it happens, no matter how stupid it sounds.

At a certain point, they might simply go along for the ride and, with an apparently saintly acceptance, yield to the state of *not knowing*. We should all be so chilled.

Even if your increasingly forgetful wife has never been a joiner, she may get into things like an exercise program at the local seniors' centre. This will do wonders for her mind and body.

Don't condescend. Just when you think they've lost it completely, they'll remember some obscure fact from *your* past that *you'd* forgotten.

Or wished you had.

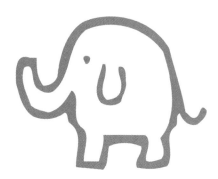

When grandad tells the waitress he wants her to have his children (often in more colourful language), apologise to her and forgive him. Dementia sufferers lose the ability to censor themselves.

And don't beat yourself up for finding this stuff funny. It *is* funny. Consider your laughter a small reward for looking after them.

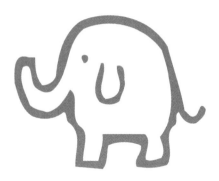

It's hard not to feel wounded when dad yells, hits, kicks or even bites you, but remember he's simply angry about something and it's not personal. If you can't figure out what it is, it's best just to give him some space.

And try not to bite back.

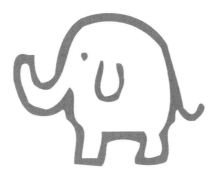

If they struggle with utensils, prepare finger food for their meals.

Saves on the washing up too!

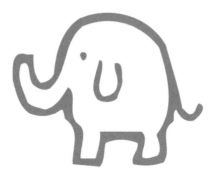

One minute, your once sharp husband will know what to do with his dental floss and in the next ask what such a strange thing is used for. Accept these cognitive glitches like you would a day with both sunshine and rain, and you will be a happier camper.

When you're out for a drive, they may feel compelled to read the street signs out loud, so let them. It's their way of making sense of the world and showing off a little at the same time. Even if no one, including your five-year-old, is impressed.

Symptoms of senility can be amplified by a house move or a partner being away or dying. So, use other familiar things, places, people to shore up their sense of wellbeing.

Every few hours, ask them if they need to go to the toilet or, better yet, take them. And watch for signs that they need to go, like pulling down their pants in the middle of the street.

But don't be grossed out when they have to start wearing nappies.

You used to wear them! You just don't remember.

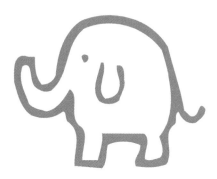

When they get to the nappy stage, put a large plastic bag or some memory foam over the car seat (or their regular chair) with a tucked-in towel on top. In case of leakage, you won't have to replace the entire seat.

If they ask why there's a towel over their seat, tell them you spilled some water and don't want them to get wet.

As their dementia progresses, they will sleep *a lot*. Use the opportunity to squeeze in a tiny bit of your own life.

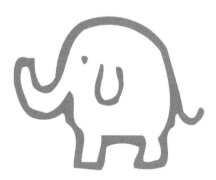

If they move in with you, know that it's like having a toddler who weighs as much as you do. It ain't gonna be easy. But try to act like it's a privilege, not a chore, even if you don't always feel that way. You're setting an example for your own kids, who might have to wrestle *you* to the bathroom one of these days.

If you set them up in a room in your place, bring some of their own stuff, even if it's falling apart. Their ratty old blanket and moth-eaten lampshade will give them more comfort than brand-new-everything from Ikea.

Encourage them to write down the things they need to 'remember'.

But don't rely on their notes, which can get lost, misread,

flushed away or eaten.

Remember those questions your four-year-old asked, like why we only dress up on Halloween and whether dogs can fly? Well, be prepared to be asked again by your eighty-year-old dad.

And remember that there's no such thing as a stupid question, only stupid answers.

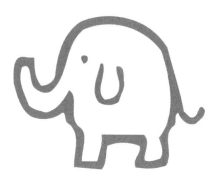

Approach their bedtime the way you would with a child: with soft tones, gentle music, a night light or two.

And if they want a teddy bear, give them one. Even yours.

You can never contradict a dementia sufferer's answers because they won't remember the question.

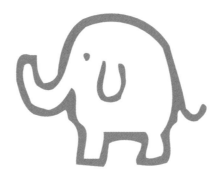

And don't contradict their perceptions of time. If they think they spent a day at the beach instead of an hour, does it matter?

Keep them playing memory and cognitive games like crosswords as long as they can. Even when they get most of the answers wrong.

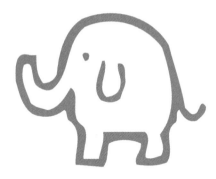

And play them yourself to keep your own noodle sharp.

If you make them uncomfortable about telling you they forget, they'll hide it when they do. And it becomes a danger when it's about whether they've taken their medication or eaten that day.

Don't let them watch violent or scary TV shows – they can't always tell the difference between drama and reality. Do you really want them thinking *Nightmare on Elm Street* is their new address?

To understand what they're going through, try to imagine being dropped in the middle of a completely unfamiliar house among total strangers every day.

So, be kind.

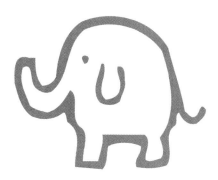

Dementia can be a great disinhibitor. Don't be surprised if they acquire a sudden fondness for manga porn.

And let them indulge, as long as they don't share it with the kids.

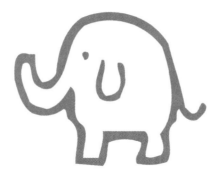

Don't think of their broken trains of thought as derailments but as detours on alternative tracks, taking you places you never expected to go.

What they're going through is the reverse of what Bill Murray went through in *Groundhog Day*. When they wake up they'll have no idea what happened yesterday, so they can't learn from it. Rather than becoming wiser, they'll become more like a child.

Don't be surprised if mum gets upset when something disrupts her daily routine. Routine gives her day the shape that her memory can no longer define.

Try not to let it get to you the first time they don't know who you are.

The head may forget but, deep down, the heart still knows.

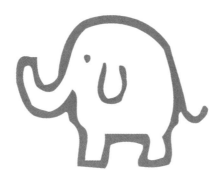

If it's your partner who's losing it, accept that you will feel a lot of anger. They vowed to be with you 'till death us do part', and now that their brain is departing it feels like a betrayal. Once you understand this, it can be a bit easier to cope.

But don't feel guilty if you're still angry – even after they're gone.

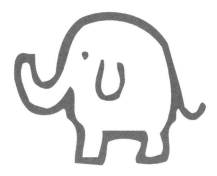

Brain deterioration from dementia can prompt sufferers to make unfounded accusations, so don't get upset when dad says, 'You stole my vacuum cleaner!' Just find the vacuum cleaner and show him.

Unless you stole it.

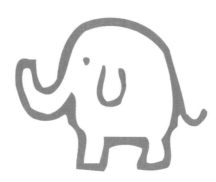

Revel in the absurdity of their strange observations and *non sequiturs*. They probably won't get what you're laughing at anyway, and think *you're* the loon.

Keep them connected to the community. Trips to their favourite café or the library or the pub where they'll see vaguely familiar faces can work wonders.

Encourage their friends to stay in touch. Sometimes it's easy to walk away, but most people will be happy to visit or call. All they need is a little nudge.

And if you have to, bribe them with the promise of a meal.

Drinks. Cash.

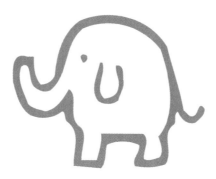

One of the hardest things to put up with is their resentment of you taking care of them.

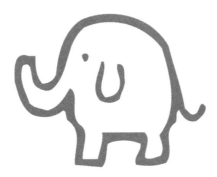

But what's even harder is your *own* resentment. It's never going to make sense – especially if *they're* the parent, *you're* the child. So, learn to forgive yourself while you're learning to forgive them.

Their stories may become more and more absurd, such as 'I didn't give birth to you, unlike your sister . . . I found you in a pine tree.'

Or, 'The time I was abducted by aliens, your father wanted to come but they didn't like his haircut.' Just enjoy them.

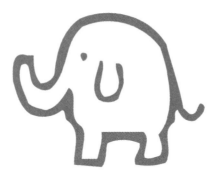

Don't be surprised when, in the midst of the haze of forgetfulness, they display the odd flash of memory brilliance. Connections in the brain sometimes sizzle before they fizzle.

At some point, their dream life and waking life seem to merge. Think of it as an opportunity to see inside someone's unedited, unorganised, untethered subconscious – the human psyche at its most liberated!

The more out-of-it she gets, the more mum may insist on staying in the house she's lived in for sixty years. But you have to balance her need for independence with the prospect of her burning the place down.

When things get to that point, tour the local care homes you can afford. Most of them are not nightmare landscapes from Hieronymus Bosch, but well-run facilities full of hardworking professionals who can save your sanity.

When you're getting them settled in care, surrender to the paperwork that will flow like a flood-swollen river.

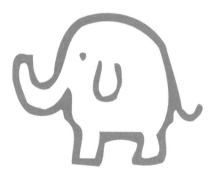

Even if it's the nicest place on the planet, they will say at some point that they want to go home. Rather than explain for the forty-seventh time that you sold the old homestead, distract them with something (a picture, a book . . . a doughnut!) that may head off a tantrum.

The further the disease progresses, the more you need to embrace the 'therapeutic lie'. If telling your dad that the house is being repainted rather than that developers have demolished it makes him feel better, then do so. His sense of wellbeing is more important than the truth.

No matter how annoying she can be and how much you secretly wish she'd fall off the perch, don't be surprised if you miss her when she's gone.

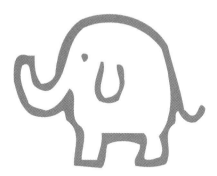

While they're still with us, tell them you love them every day.

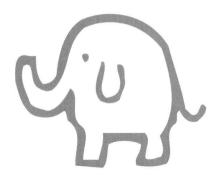